OUTBREAK!

SPANISH FLU

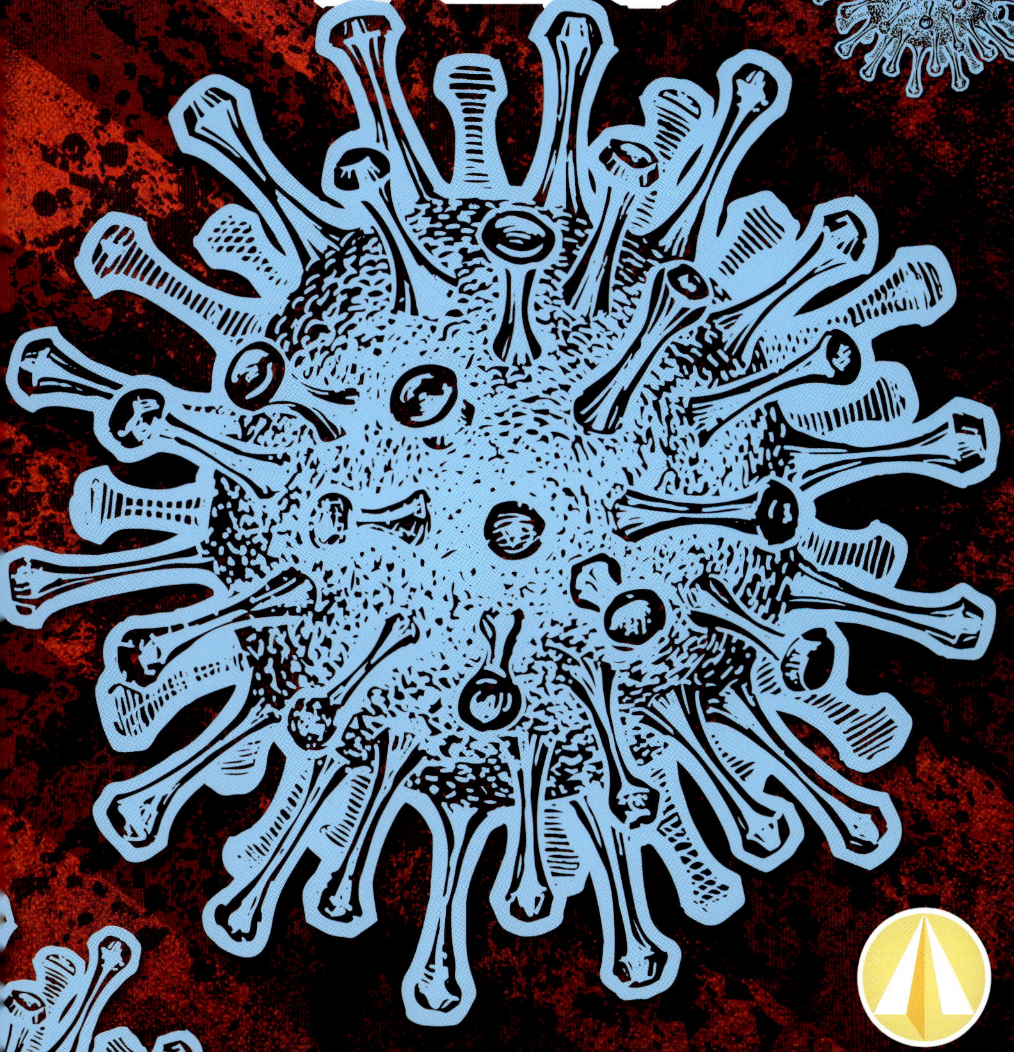

KENNY ABDO

Fly!
An Imprint of Abdo Zoom
abdobooks.com

abdobooks.com

Published by Abdo Zoom, a division of ABDO, P.O. Box 398166, Minneapolis, Minnesota 55439.

Printed in the United States of America, North Mankato, Minnesota.
102020
012021

THIS BOOK CONTAINS RECYCLED MATERIALS

Photo Credits: Alamy, AP Images, Library of Congress, newscom, Science Source, Shutterstock
Production Contributors: Kenny Abdo, Jennie Forsberg, Grace Hansen
Design Contributors: Dorothy Toth, Neil Klinepier, Laura Graphenteen

Library of Congress Control Number: 2020910904

Publisher's Cataloging-in-Publication Data

Names: Abdo, Kenny, author.
Title: Spanish Flu / by Kenny Abdo
Description: Minneapolis, Minnesota : Abdo Zoom, 2021 | Series: Outbreak! | Includes online resources and index.
Identifiers: ISBN 9781098223298 (lib. bdg.) | ISBN 9781098223991 (ebook) | ISBN 9781098224349 (Read-to-Me ebook)
Subjects: LCSH: Influenza Epidemic, 1918-1919--Juvenile literature. | Influenza viruses--Juvenile literature. | Epidemics--Juvenile literature. | Epidemics-History--Juvenile literature. | Plague--History--Juvenile literature.
Classification: DDC 614.49--dc23

TABLE OF CONTENTS

Spanish Flu 4

Symptoms.......................... 8

Source 10

Outbreak! 14

Glossary 22

Online Resources 23

Index 24

SPANISH FLU

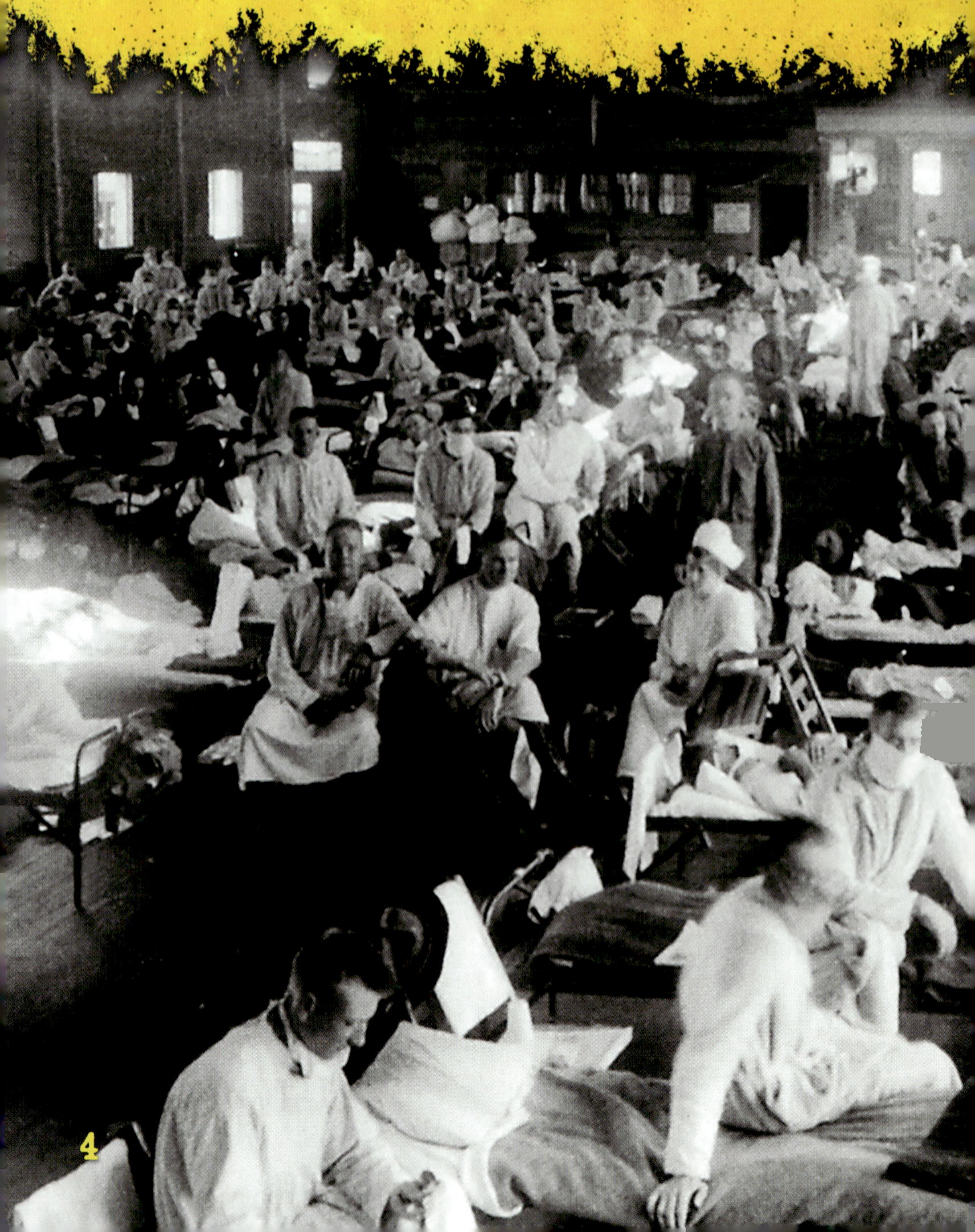

The namesake of one country, the Spanish flu rocked the entire world for more than a year.

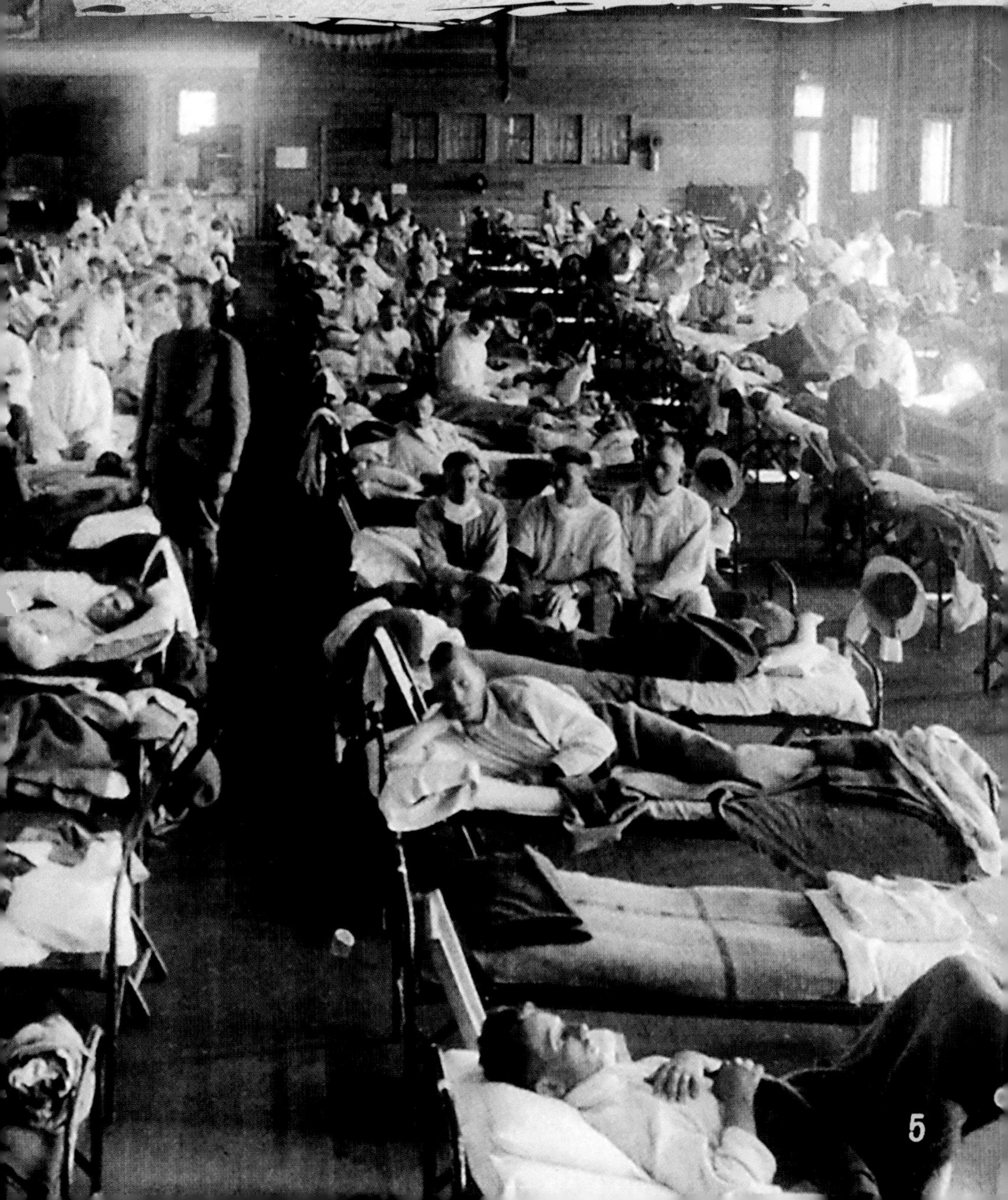

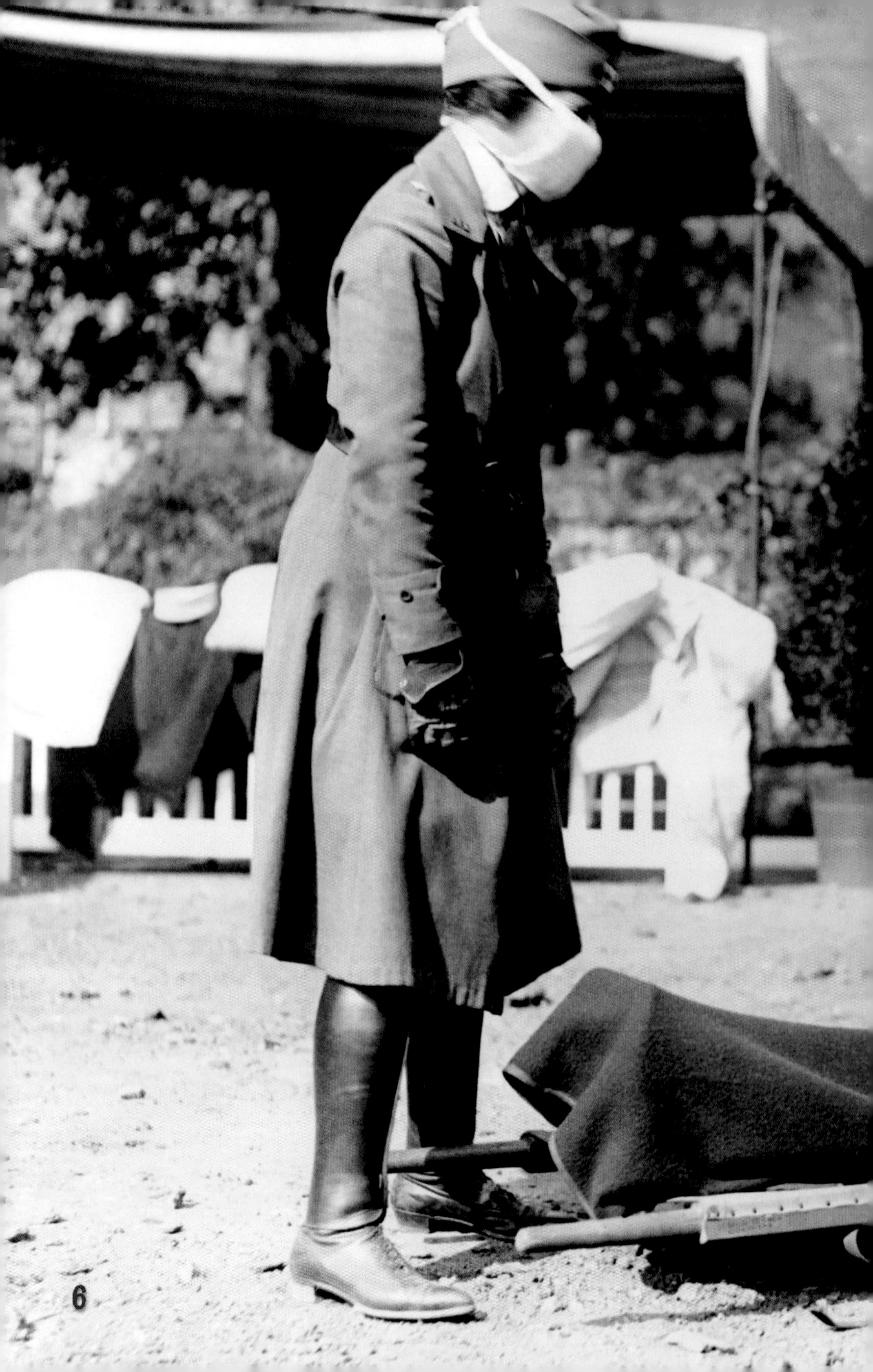

Between wars being fought and the spread of the Spanish flu, 1918 was a year of unrest and sadness.

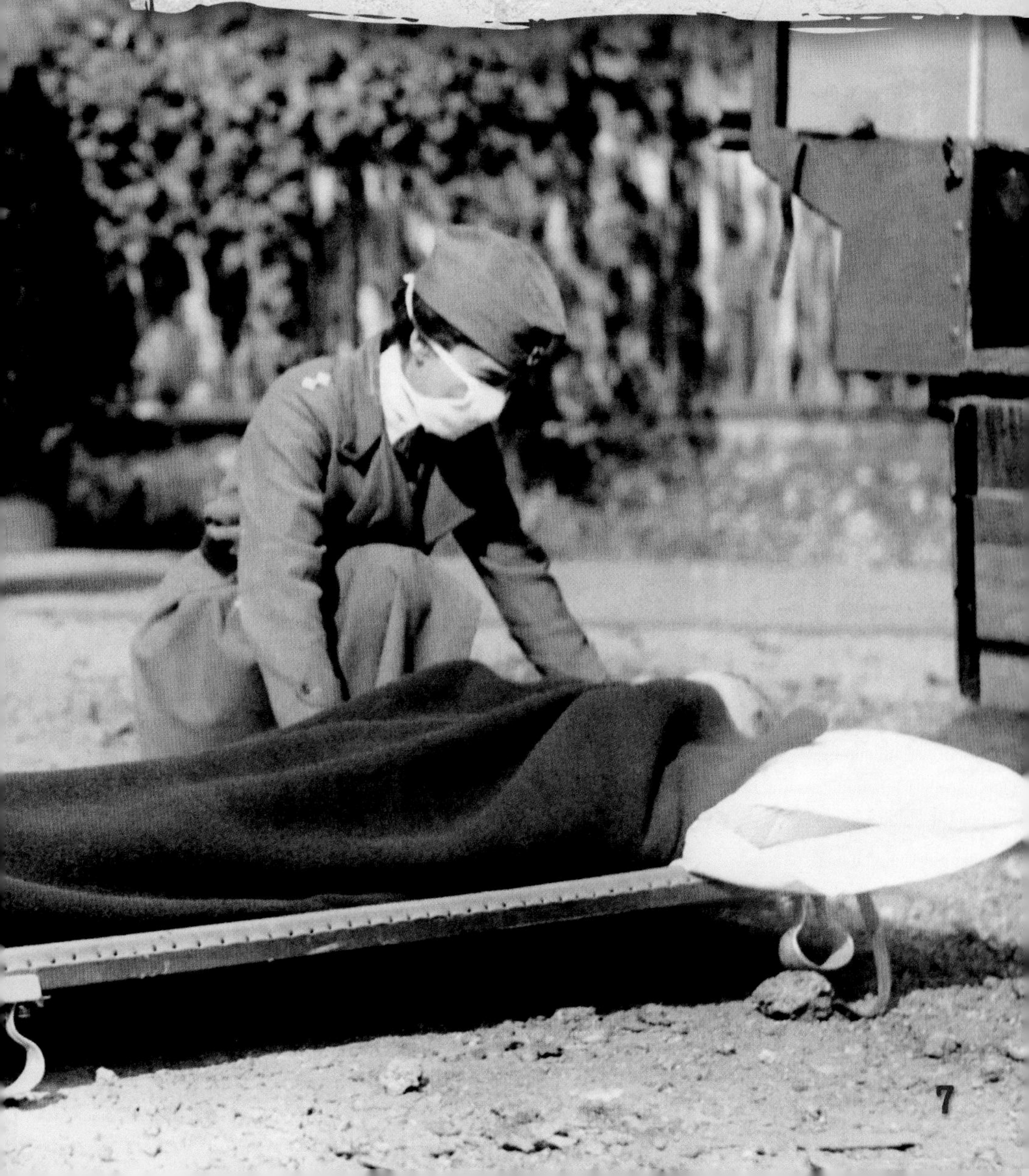

SYMPTOMS

The Spanish flu began with normal flu **symptoms**. People experienced chills, fever, and tiredness. Those **infected** usually recovered after just a few days.

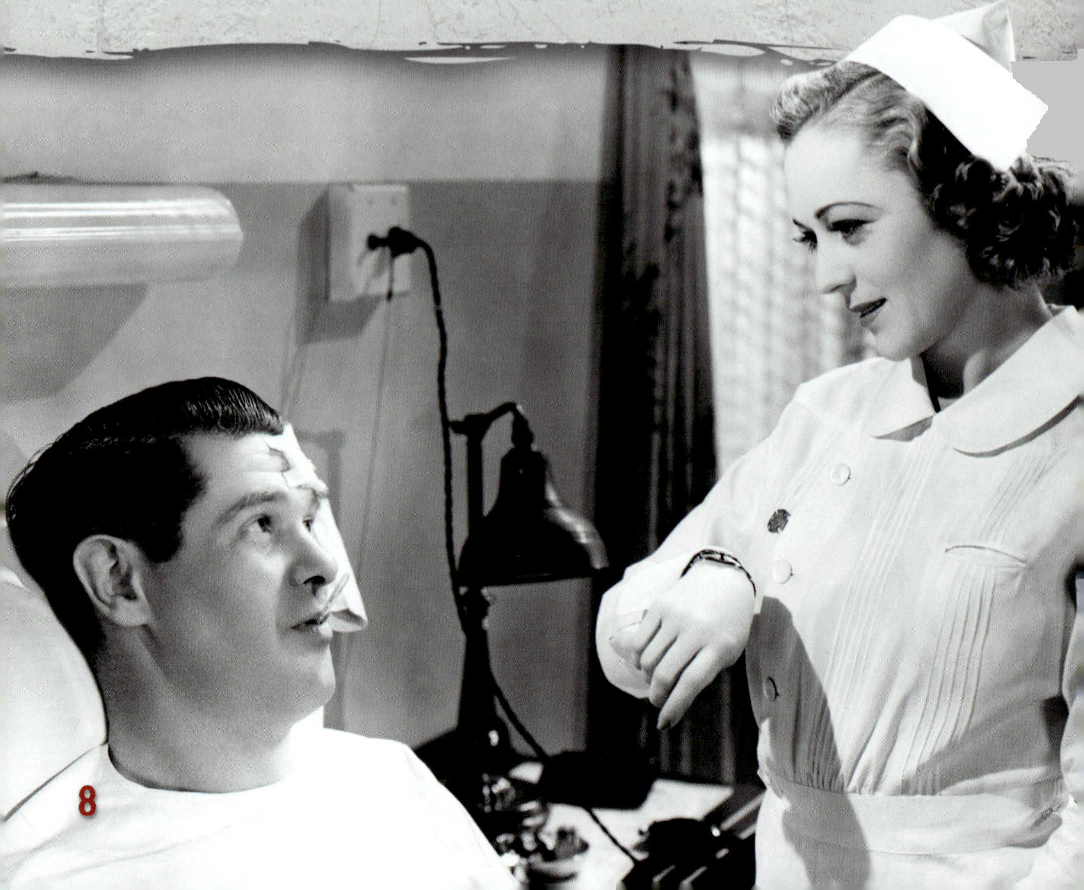

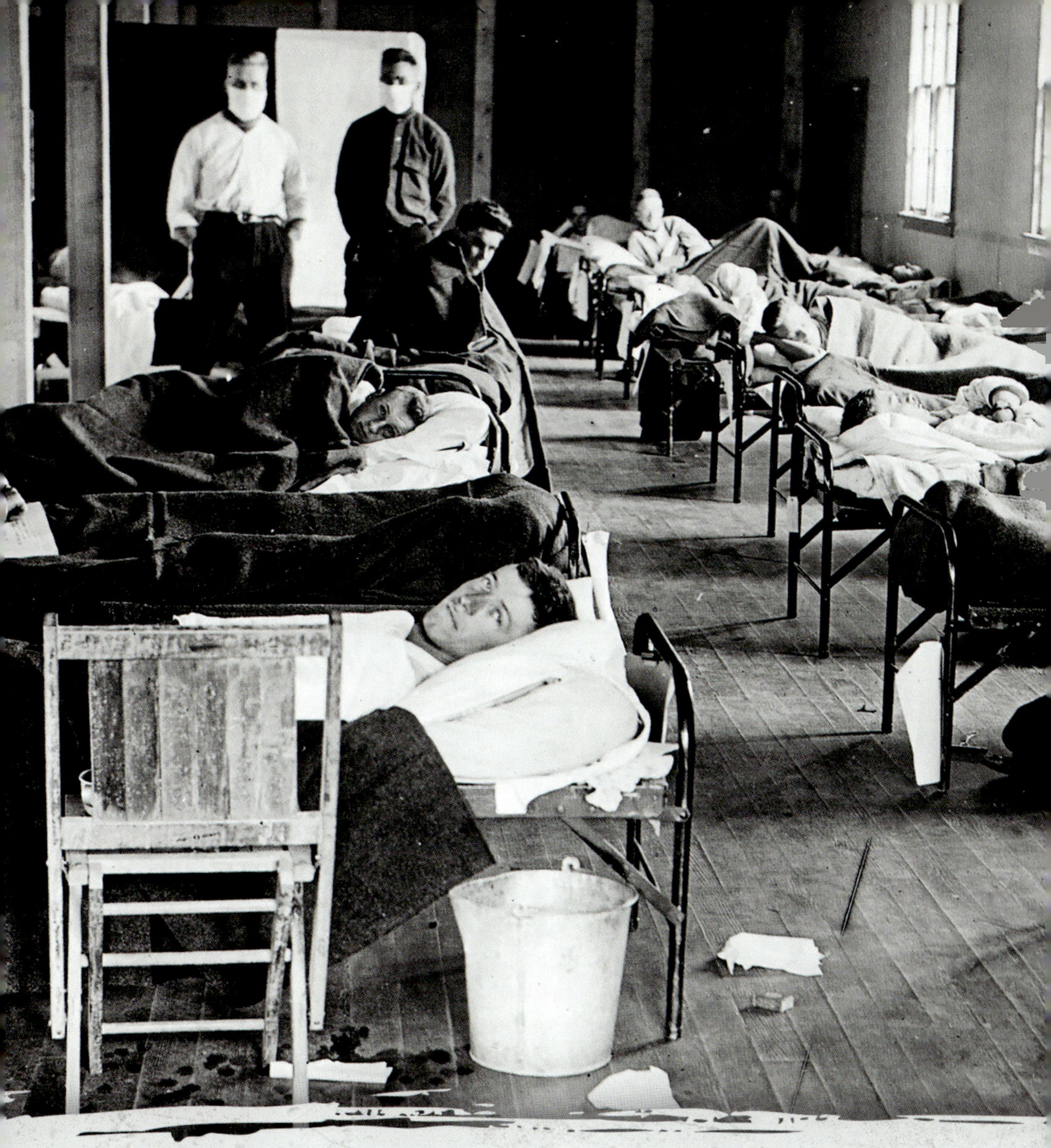

A second wave of the illness brought more serious **symptoms**. People died within hours of showing symptoms. Their skin turned blue. Their lungs filled with fluid, suffocating them.

SOURCE

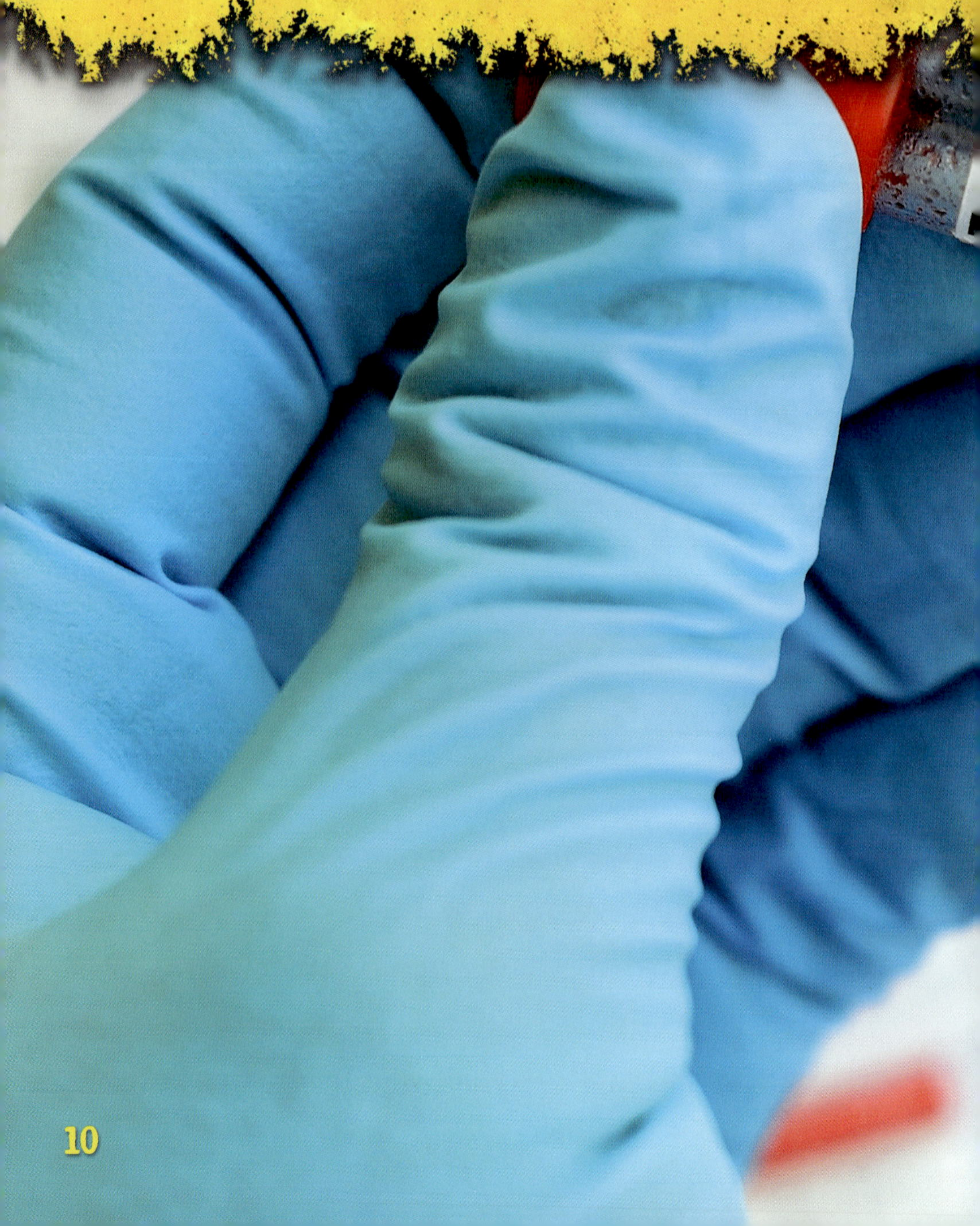

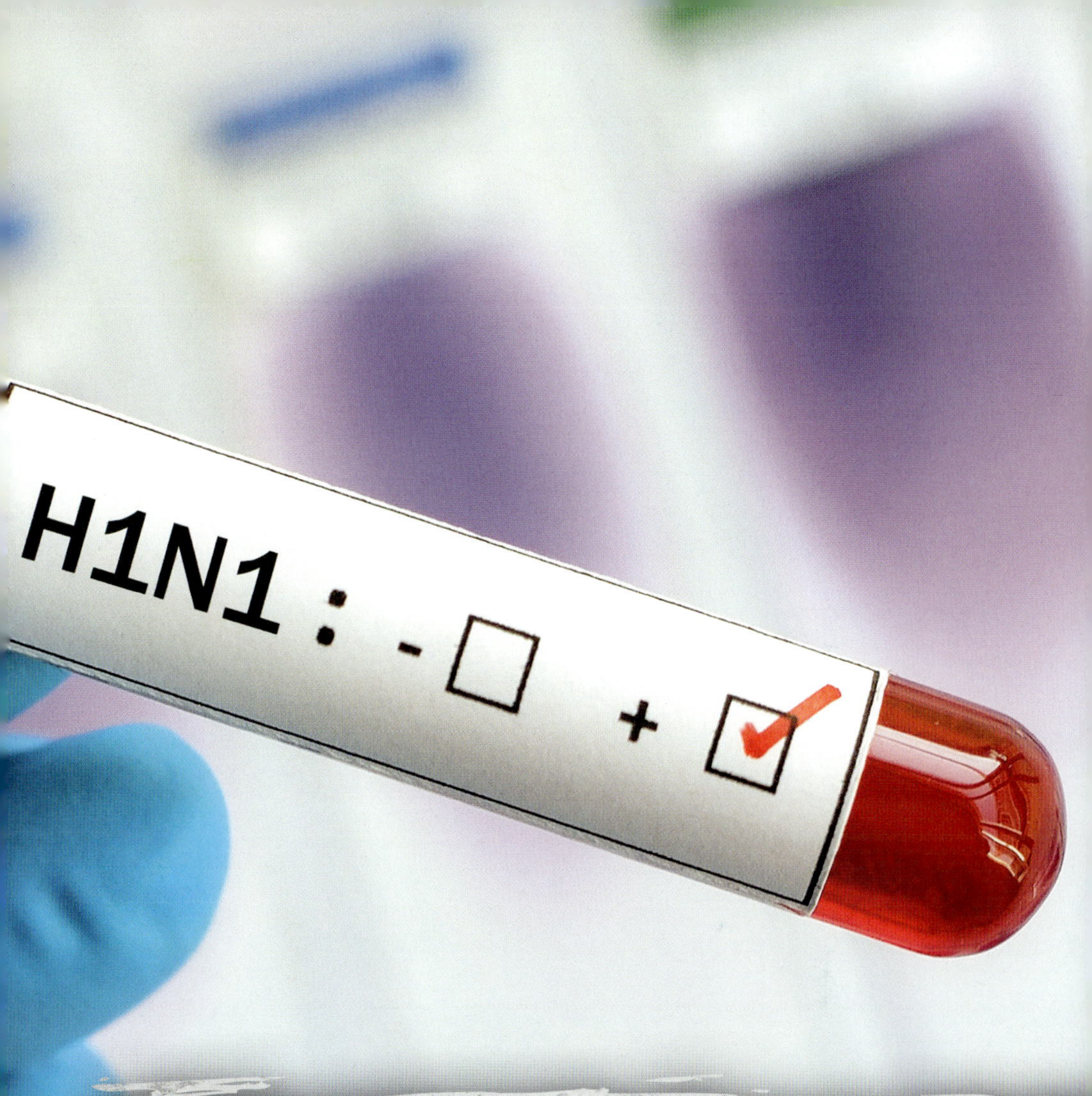

H1N1 is a virus strain that started in pigs. Those who caught it would suffer a flu that varied from mild to deadly. Scientists still are not sure which country the virus originated in.

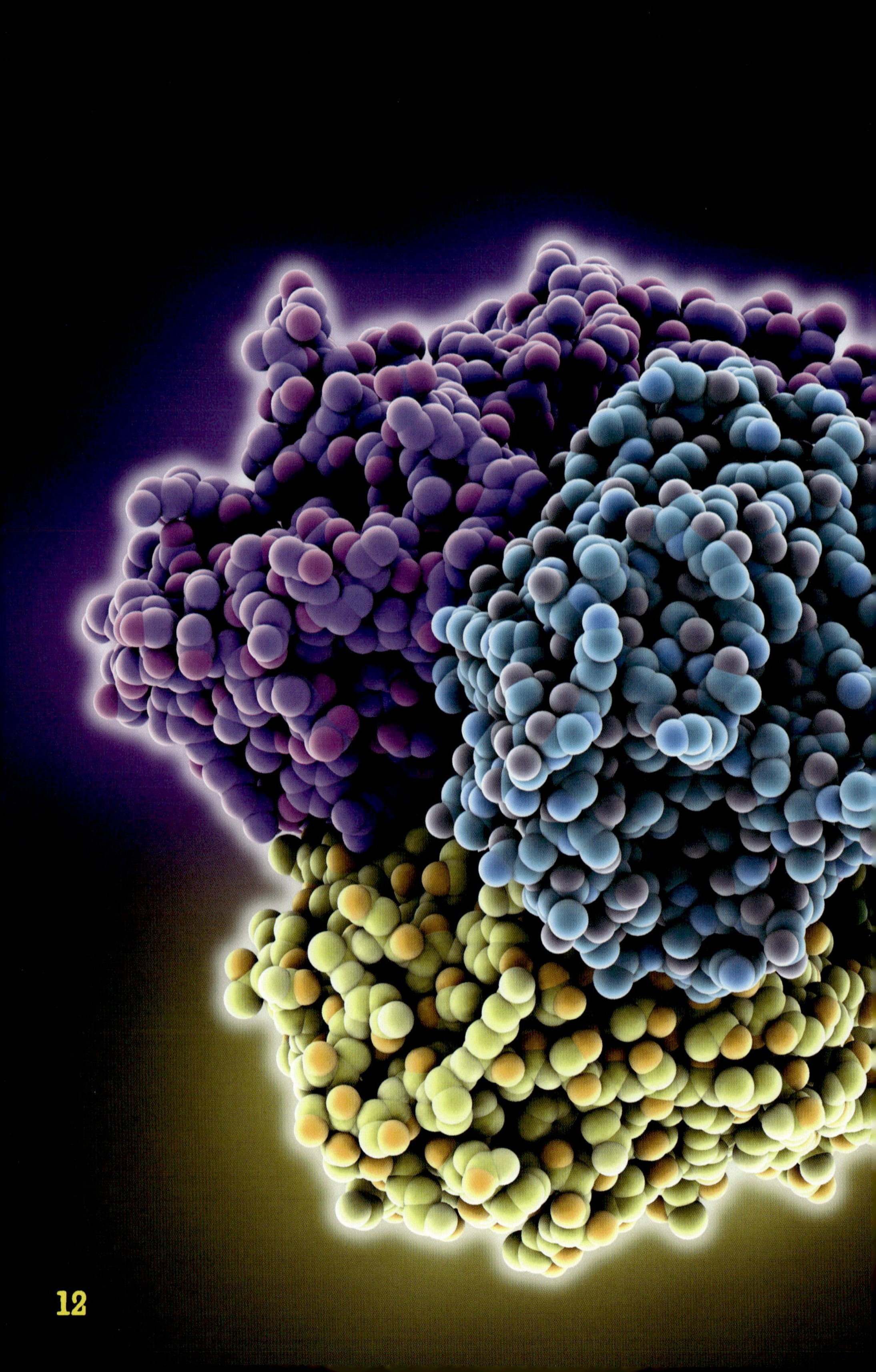

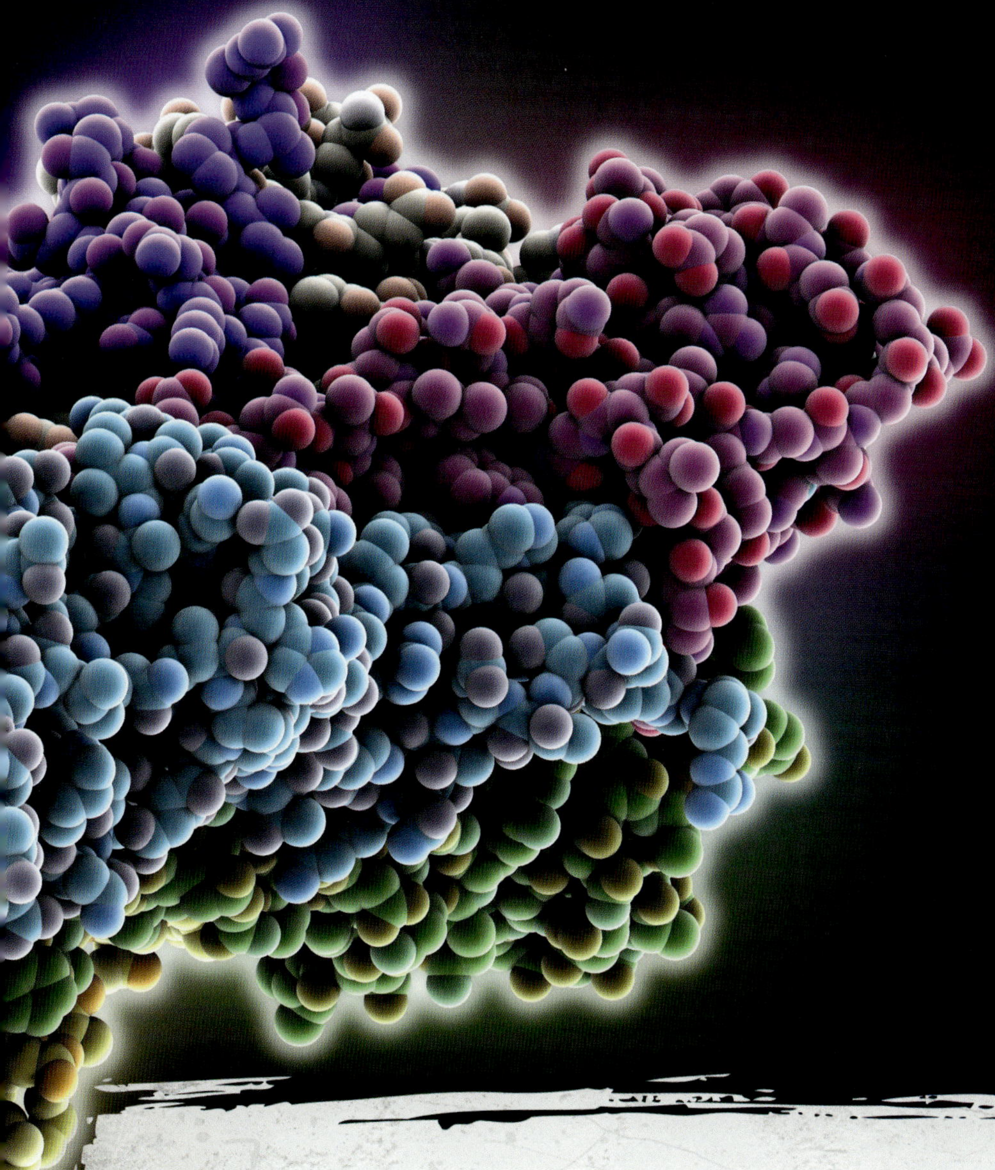

The Spanish flu was born from the H1N1 influenza A virus. By 1918, it had evolved to be deadlier and more **contagious**.

OUTBREAK!

During World War I, countries involved were in a media **blackout**. One of the few places reporting its flu cases was Spain. Because Spain was reporting flu cases, the illness was named after the country.

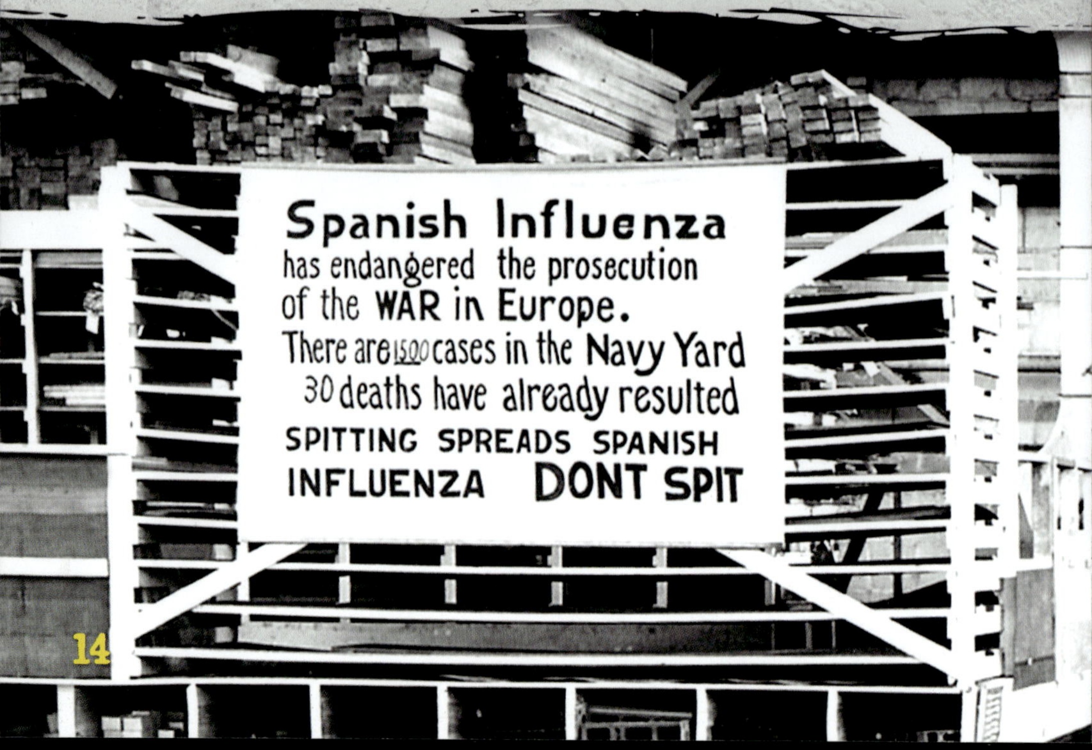

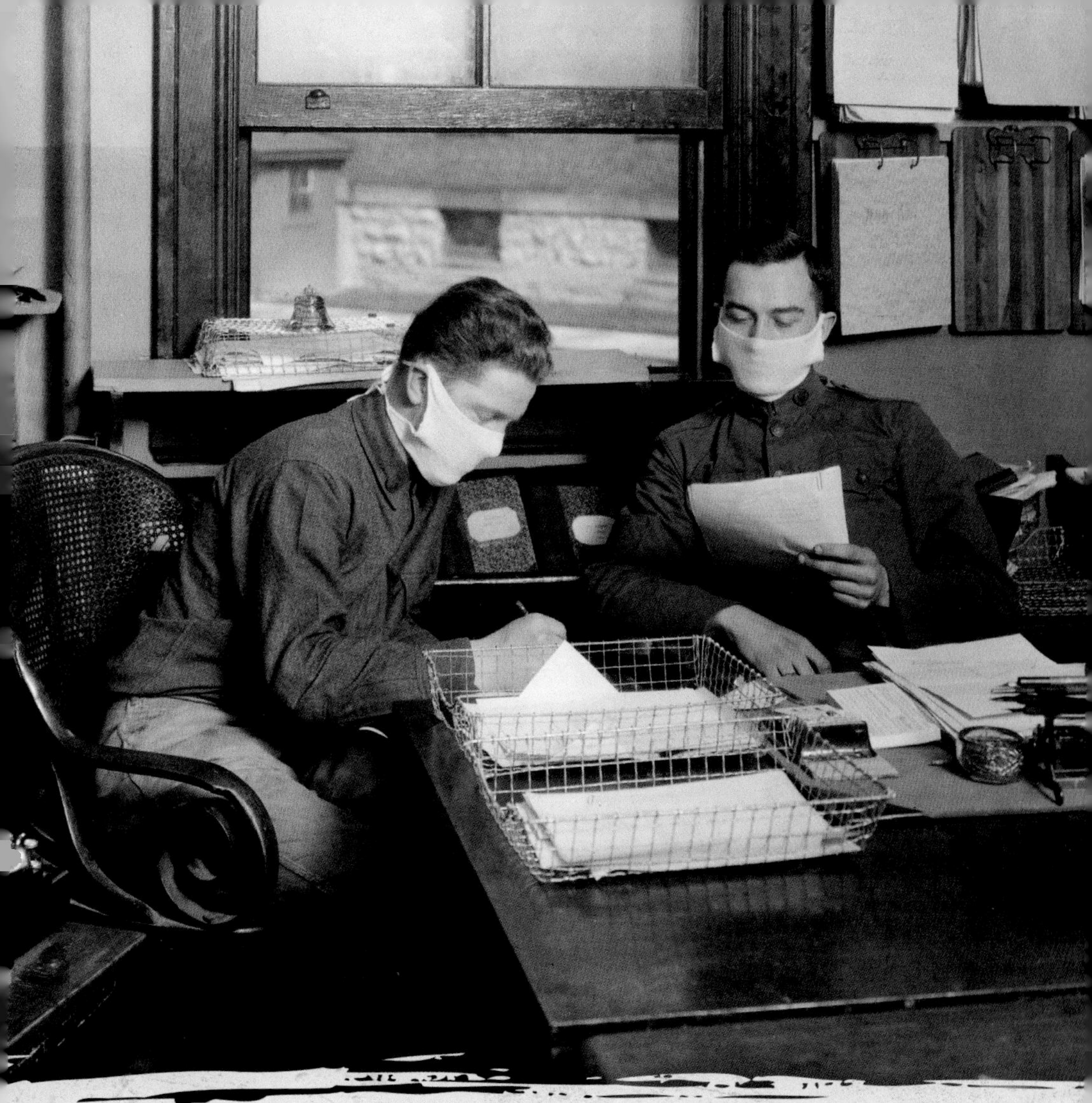

The Spanish flu was first mentioned in the US in April 1918. There were 18 cases and three deaths at Fort Riley in Kansas. Reports of the flu showed it spread throughout the US, Europe, and Asia.

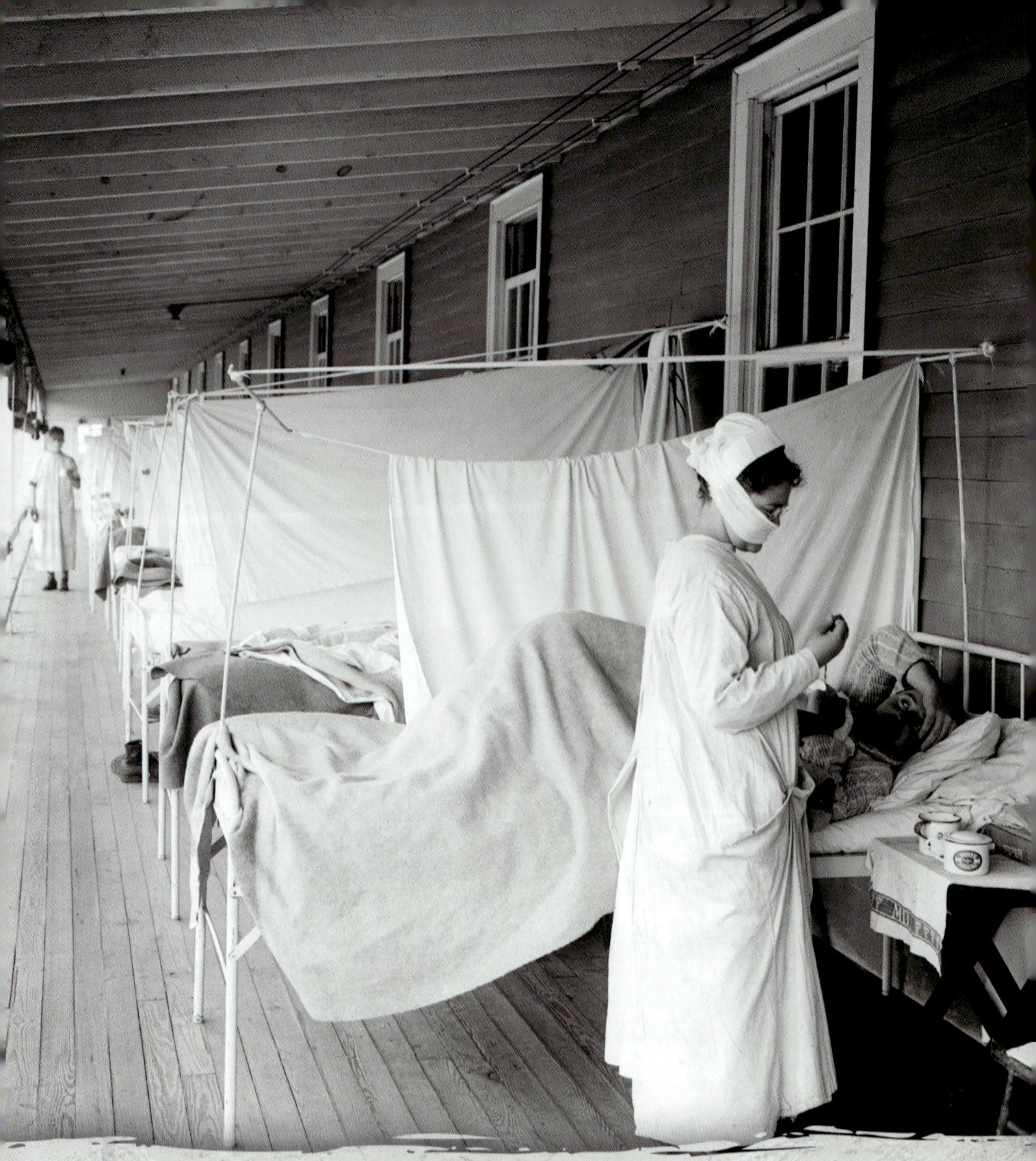

The second wave of the virus hit in September. By October, it had grown into a **pandemic**. It killed an estimated 195,000 Americans in that month alone.

Quarantines and hygiene education programs were put into place by November. Citizens in San Francisco were fined $5 if they were caught in public without face masks.

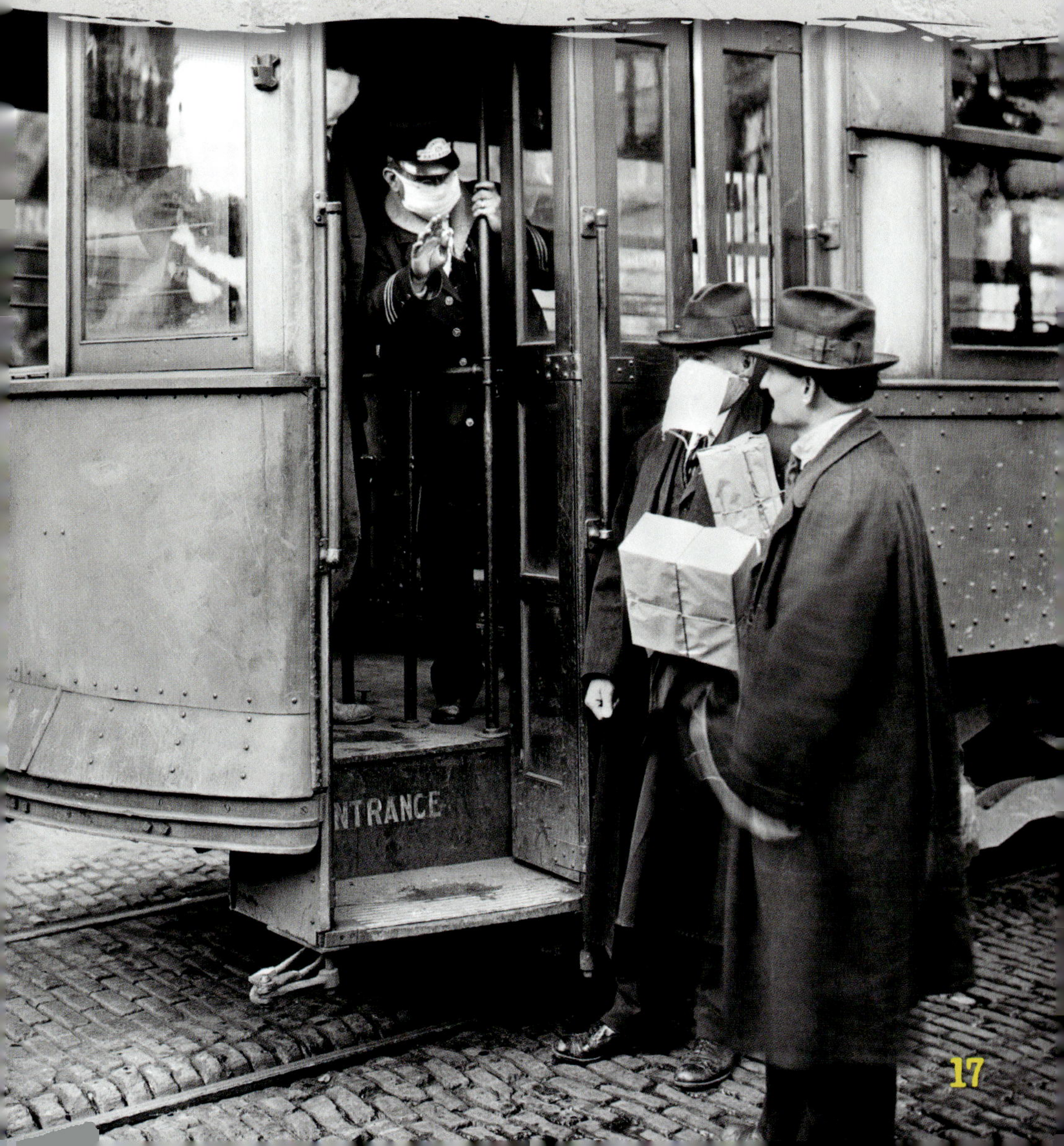

More than 500 million people became **infected** with the virus. That was one-third of the world's population at the time.

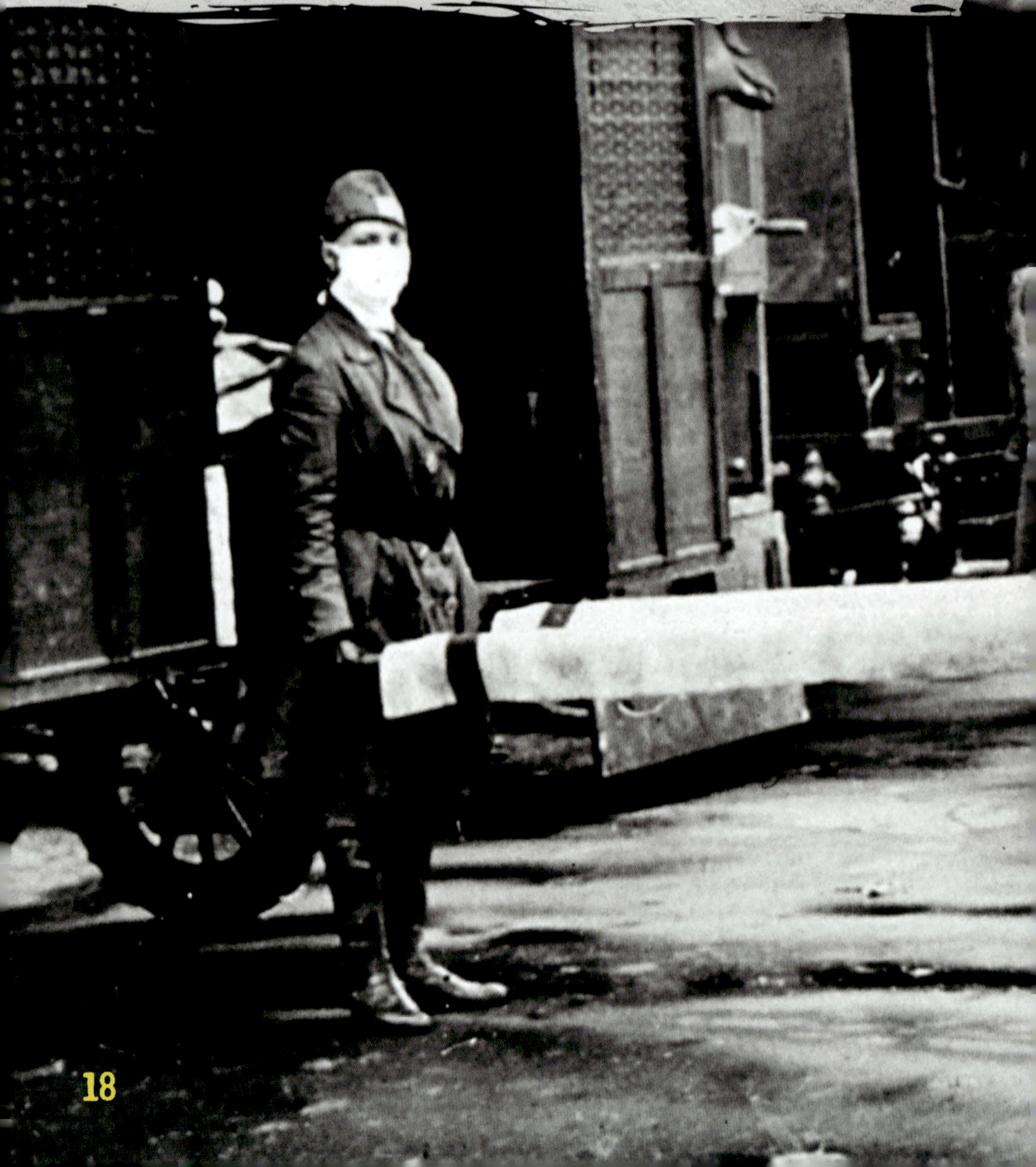

The number of deaths is estimated to be more than 50 million worldwide.

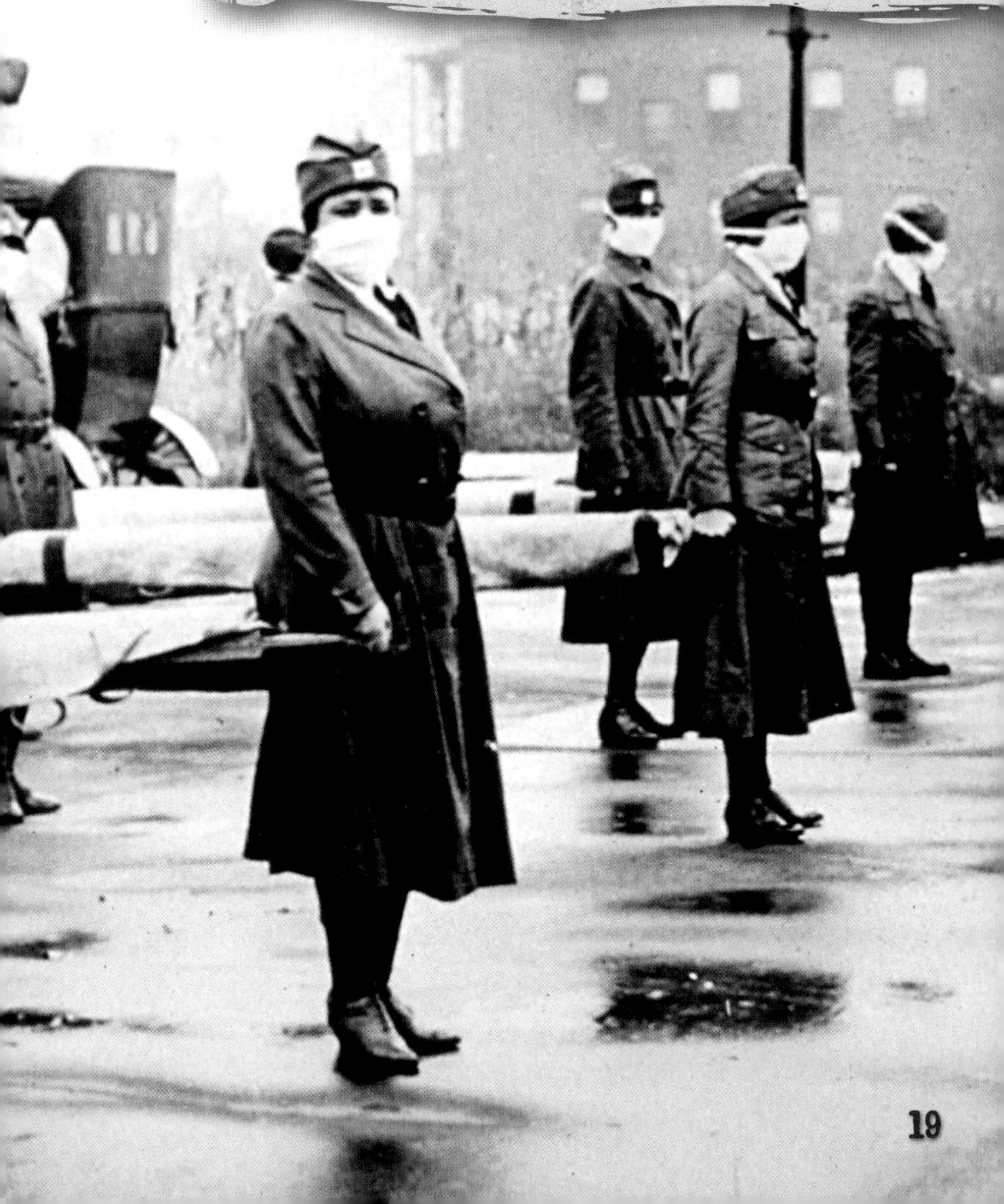

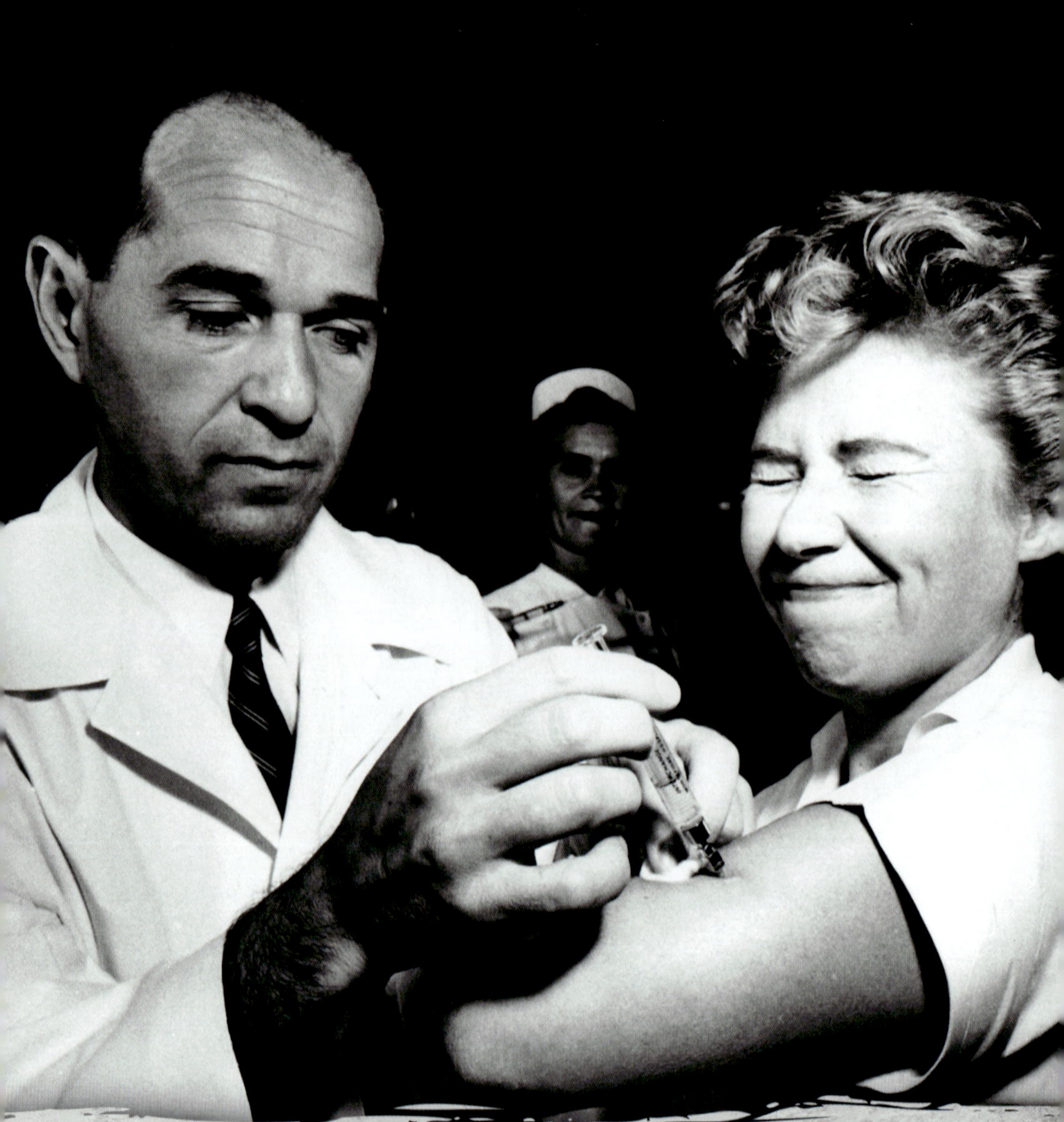

The third wave hit in January of 1919. The Spanish Flu **pandemic** came to an end in the summer of 1919. Those who were **infected** had either died or developed **immunity**.

By 2005, scientists had learned more about the Spanish flu. However, flu viruses often change. So, scientists have to work hard to keep the viruses from triggering another **pandemic**.

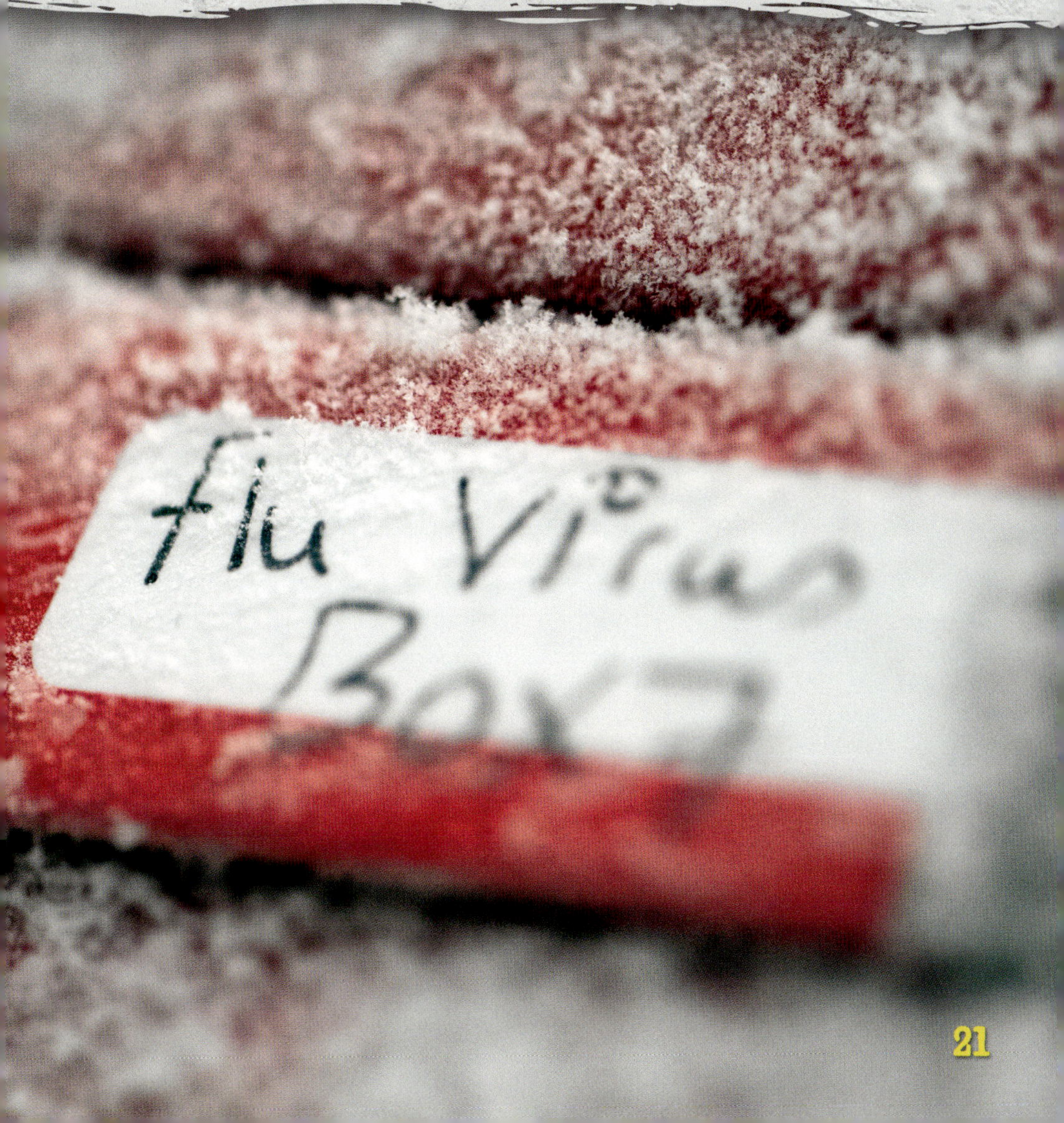

GLOSSARY

blackout – removing the news of a certain topic for a specific reason.

contagious – a disease that spreads from person to person by direct or indirect contact.

immunity – resistance to infections and diseases.

infect – to spread germs or disease to.

pandemic – a disease that spreads quickly around the world in a short amount of time.

quarantine – a period of time when sick people separate themselves from others to avoid spreading a disease.

symptoms – the signs that a person is ill or is becoming sick.

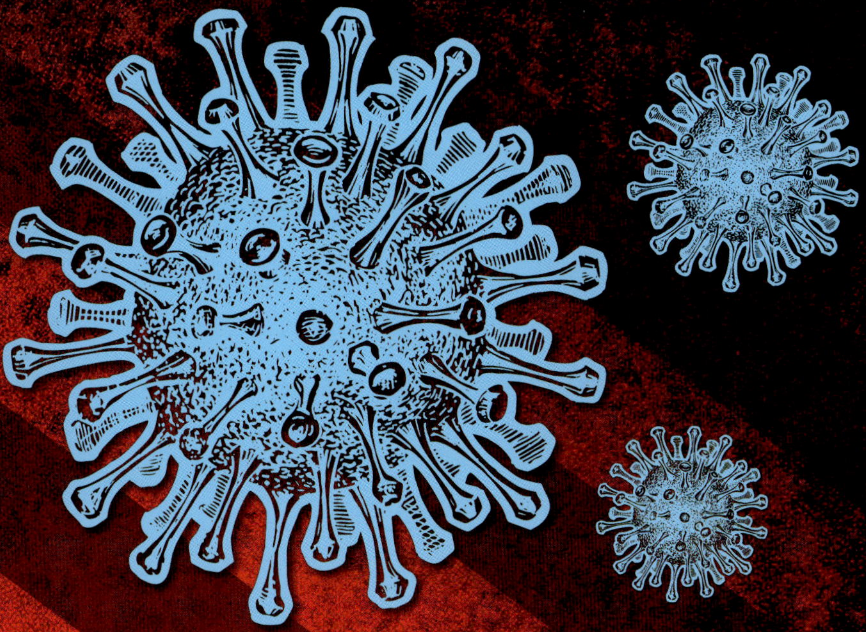

ONLINE RESOURCES

Booklinks
NONFICTION NETWORK
FREE! ONLINE NONFICTION RESOURCES

To learn more about Spanish flu, please visit **abdobooklinks.com** or scan this QR code. These links are routinely monitored and updated to provide the most current information available.

INDEX

Asia 15

Europe 15

H1N1 virus 11, 13

media 14

prevention 17

research 21

signs 8, 9, 11

Spain 5, 14

spread 13, 15, 16, 18, 19

symptoms 8, 9, 11

United States 15, 16, 17

World War I 7, 14